I0094724

A Better Normal for Body Confidence

Your Guide to Rediscovering Intimacy After Cancer

Tess Devèze

Published in Australia by ConnectAble Therapies Pty Ltd.

1510 Mills Road, Glen Forrest WA 6071, Australia
Copyright © 2023 Tess Devèze
All rights reserved.

No part of this publication may be reproduced, stored in a retrieval
system, or transmitted, in any form or by any means, electronic,
mechanical, photocopying, recording or otherwise, without the prior
permission of the author & creator.

This book is sold subject to the condition that it shall not, by way of
trade or otherwise be lent, re-sold, hired out or otherwise circulated
without the creator's prior consent in any form of binding or cover
other than that in which it is purchased.

Disclaimer: All care has been taken in the preparation of the
information herein, but no responsibility can be accepted by the author
for any damages resulting from the misinterpretation of this work. The
content in this book shall not be used as an alternative to seeking
professional and clinical advice.

For more information see www.connectabletherapies.com

ISBN: 978-0-6453101-2-2

CONTENTS

WHY I WROTE THIS BOOK

Hello! It's so wonderful to meet you. I'm Tess.

I thought before we get into the more 'intimate' details, I'd introduce myself and let you know what this book is about.

I was diagnosed with stage-three breast cancer in 2018, at the age of 36. At the time of my diagnosis, I'd been working in the sexuality sector for years. Over the years since my cancer diagnosis and endless treatments, only twice did a healthcare professional voluntarily bring up the topic of sexuality and only one booklet was recommended to me (which I had to go and find myself). The lack of information and support on this topic, both during and after treatments, was painfully noticeable.

Why aren't more resources available? Why are we so afraid to talk about this essential aspect of our lives?

First and foremost, I'm an occupational therapist (OT). What's an OT, I hear you ask? We are functional therapists and use specific approaches to promote independence and participation in 'occupations' which are any kind of meaningful life activity that occupies us. OT's help you do the day-to-day activities that you need and want to do, as best you can. This may include self-care tasks (shower, dressing, toileting), work related (vocational) tasks, social or community activities…and may also include sex!

My clinical experience is mostly in sexuality - during and after cancer treatments, brain-injury, neurological conditions, and those living with disability. Before moving solely to sexuality for people with cancer, disability and chronic illness, most of my work was in private and public hospitals across Australia, working in neurological rehabilitation. I love neuroscience, and most of my work is based on neurological concepts.

Other than having cancer and being a sexuality OT, I also work with sexuality and self-development pioneers 'Curious Creatures', based in Melbourne Australia. I've facilitated hundreds of workshops online and face to face for nearing a decade, teaching consent, better intimacy and communication skills. I've seen thousands of people's lives change through a deeper understanding of sexual intimacy.

Lastly, I've also studied somatic sexological bodywork at the Institute of Somatic Sexology. This training has given me a deeper understanding of how libido, pleasure, arousal and orgasmicity (cool word huh?) work on a physiological, neurological, and psychological level. These learnings form an essential part of this book.

Even with all my training, I've struggled. If you're struggling too, you're not alone (even if it doesn't get spoken about).

But it's not just about me. The contents of this book are also guided by you. I have a Facebook group 'Intimacy and Cancer' with thousands of people - all cancers, all genders - from over 49 countries, who share and support each other on this topic. My one-on-one clients have also been a huge source of learning, generously sharing their experiences.

It's been almost two years since releasing 'A Better Normal; Your Guide to Rediscovering Intimacy After Cancer', and the positive feedback I have personally been receiving from readers has been at times overwhelming. I am humbled, amazed and inspired by the impact and influence this book has had for those out there suffering.

But cancer treatments are *haaaaaard*, and so is reading! I wanted to know how I could reach more people, change more lives for the better through the contents in this book. In answer to that question, I've created the 'A Better Normal' mini-book *series*. It's a number of bite-sized treatment or side-effect specific mini-books, to help cancer patients and their loved ones maintain and grow connection, intimacy and sexuality. Each mini-book is created from the information in 'A Better Normal; Your Guide to Rediscovering Intimacy After Cancer', but broken down into simple, easy-to-read guides relative to your very specific needs, because often during and after treatments committing to a 300-page book feels overwhelming or is simply not possible.

Books in the 'A Better Normal' mini-book series are:

- 'A Better Normal for **Libido**; Your Guide to Rediscovering Intimacy After Cancer'
- 'A Better Normal for **Vaginal Dryness & Pain**; Your Guide to Rediscovering Intimacy After Cancer'
- 'A Better Normal for **Body Confidence**; Your Guide to Rediscovering Intimacy After Cancer'
- 'A Better Normal for **Chemotherapy**; Your Guide to Rediscovering Intimacy After Cancer'
- 'A Better Normal for **Hormone Therapy**; Your Guide to Rediscovering Intimacy After Cancer'
- 'A Better Normal for **Fatigue**; Your Guide to Rediscovering Intimacy After Cancer'

- 'A Better Normal for **Changes In Erection**; Your Guide to Rediscovering Intimacy After Cancer'
- 'A Better Normal for **Radiotherapy**; Your Guide to Rediscovering Intimacy After Cancer'
- 'A Better Normal for **Pain**; Your Guide to Rediscovering Intimacy After Cancer'

Or if you're after all of the above information (and more) in one place, the all-in-one book 'A Better Normal; Your Guide to Rediscovering Intimacy After Cancer' has everything you need.

If you end up with several mini-books in the series, that's pretty normal, as we don't have only one side-effect (geez, wouldn't that be nice!), and we can have the same side-effect from more than one treatment (like fatigue, or changes in libido). Cancer treatments impact us differently, which is why some books in this series are side-effect specific, and others treatment specific. So you can pick and choose what is most relevant for you and where you're at. You'll also notice that some mini-books have repeated information in them. That's because some information is essential and helpful, regardless of what your side-effect or treatment is (like the communication tips, or ways to gently reconnect with yourself or a partner).

The most important thing you can learn from this book is that you're not alone and you're not broken. There's nothing wrong with you if you're struggling. It's normal to find this situation tough. This isn't one-size-fits-all advice. All bodies are unique, every relationship is different, and everyone experiences relationships, connection, pleasure and desire in their own way. You're the expert on you! Just as cancer is different for everyone, so are the connections we have with ourselves and those around us.

Lastly, this book is for all human beings, regardless of gender, lifestyle, orientation, ability, ethnicity, age, or relationship dynamic. Although every person with cancer is unique, we have one thing in common: no matter who we are or what we are going through, we're all worthy of love and connection.

Now, let's get started on making your 'new normal', a 'better normal'.

1. KEY TERMS EXPLAINED

Sexuality vs sex

The word 'sexuality' is an umbrella term which yes includes the functional activity of sex, but also includes relationships, connections, affection, dating, pleasure and our overall well-being. Sexuality can be greatly affected due to cancer, but it doesn't necessarily have to stop altogether. As a sexuality educator and clinician, I know how important sexuality, connection and intimacy is to our quality of life, our resilience and coping. What could be more important!

'Sex' in this book refers to the act, or the activity you engage in with yourself and/others, and is one of the most diverse and most adaptable functional activities I can think of. Yet today, it's still one of the most under-addressed topics in clinical settings. This is something I aim to change.

I also want us all to be on the same page in how we see 'sex' itself which is more than just orgasms and genital play, it's so much more. During cancer treatments and other life-altering events, you might need to temporarily let go of traditional forms of touch/sex. We can become excited, aroused, release pleasure hormones in our body from so many different ways. There are erogenous zones all over our bodies such as our inner thighs, breasts, nipples, under the armpits, the neck, earlobes, feet and many more depending on your body. Orgasms, engorgement, ejaculation, becoming 'hard' or 'wet', these don't need to be your goal, but can also be experienced in more than one way. Pleasure, enjoyment, arousal, excitation and connection, that is where the fun can also be. Pleasure is pleasurable and our whole body can be pleasured!

Desire vs arousal

Desire (the wanting) I use interchangeably with libido. Desire/libido are the experience of *wanting* sex and pleasure. Desire has many words that can be used, such as lust, sex-drive, and essentially all refer to that *want* we have.

Arousal is the way our body responds when it's in pleasure, the changes in our body that show us we are in fact, enjoying and excited. Things like increased sensitivity, maybe we become wet, maybe we become hard, our heart rate increases, we breathe heavier and more.

Simply put, libido = wanting, and arousal = enjoying.

Treatments can affect our arousal as well as our libido and knowing the difference between these can be very helpful.

The magical word, intimacy

Disconnection from yourself and others is a common side-effect of cancer treatments for so many. You're not alone in this and here I introduce you to the magical word 'intimacy'. Imagine that you having sex or being intimate again with yourself, a date or a partner/s, is the goal or the prize. That prize is on the other side of a river, and to get to it, you need to build a bridge. How can you do that? Through intimacy, through touch and the other magical word *affection*.

I've heard many times from clients and people in my support group "we don't even touch each other anymore". Not only has sex gone, but so has the *intimacy*, and are we really going to want sex without that connection?

Intimacy and affection are small giants. Tiny little things that can mean the world, and build that bridge of connection. Things like hand-holding, a good-night kiss, a good morning hug, your arm around your partner in the kitchen, cuddling on the couch, touch for the sake of touch (not as a way to 'get somewhere'), massage swaps, maybe a cheeky butt-squeeze and grin, and the big one, WORDS OF LOVE.

When you want some touch or love? Here's a few ways to ask, without that pressure of it needing to lead to sex:

How to say it out loud.
- "Hey, I'd like to be closer to you, how about a cuddle?"
- "Can we snuggle together on the couch while watching this film?"
- "You up for some hand-holding while we walk to the shop?"
- "I'm loving you right now, thought I'd share."
- "You up for some underwear-on cuddling while we fall asleep? I miss connecting with you."
- "I'd love some touch/to touch your body, would you like a massage?"
- "I'm not wanting this to lead to sex, but some kisses and cuddles would be lovely if you're feeling like some connection?"
- "I'm checking you out right now, just wanted to share."

- "I'm running a bath to relax and wind-down from the day, would you like to join me for some down-time?"

Small giant steps towards that prize.

2. BODY CHANGES & RECLAIMING CONFIDENCE

There are so many side-effects during treatments like fatigue, low mood, erection changes, and vaginal dryness. But there's also the visible effects such as loss of hair, weight changes, removed and/or replaced body parts and surgery scars. All can impact our physical appearance and the way we see ourselves.

As I write this, I have a surgery scar so large on my lower back I call it the 'shark-bite'. I have no nipple, just flat skin on a reconstructed breast that points in a different direction and is firm to touch. I have no sensation on that side of my chest, nor will I ever. I have stretch marks from weight gain and weight loss, I have patchy skin and my body doesn't function the way it used to. Here's the thing. People offer me compliments, but because I don't like my body, I simply don't believe them. You could tell me I'm beautiful a thousand times a day and it would be water off a duck's back. The changes to our body change the way we see ourselves which then influences the way we *feel* about ourselves. Because I don't believe you, I *won't* believe you.

The way towards us starting to believe the truth (that we

are beautiful) is to create a shift in how we feel about ourselves. So, here's 10 ways to kick-start that process.

1. Switch.

Avoid marketing and media which is designed to make us feel ugly so we buy their products. What marketing tells us we should think 'beautiful' is, is completely unachievable and unrealistic for most humans (hence the gazillion dollar 'beauty industry'). Throughout our lives we're constantly told we're not beautiful enough, that we're not good enough, so we buy the things we're told will help. It's awful, it's everywhere and it can cause or contribute to poor mental health such as depression and anxiety. Take a look at the social media, magazines, even the TV shows you watch/are exposed to, and see if you can shift towards things that have realistic and un-shaming portrayals of human diversity and human beauty. Ask around, it's out there.

2. Health.

Eat well & Exercise. I know, it's so hard (especially on treatments), but you want to feel good in yourself and getting movement day to day and eating better can help you achieve that. It can be tough, but you've faced cancer, you can do anything. Even starting with 5-10 minutes of walking a day, switching a few sugar snacks with healthier ones or trying non-alcoholic beer/wine. Baby-steps.

3. Clothes.

Wear clothing that *feels* good. If you can't wear your old clothes anymore, put them away and get new ones. If fashion is meaningful to you, it's worth the investment. If buying a new wardrobe is not affordable, alternative options are second-hand/thrift stores, websites where you can rent clothing for those dressy occasions, or find friends with a similar body shape you can borrow off (or even get hand-me-downs from!).

And watch out for behaviour changes. If you find yourself dressing differently (baggier clothes, plain darker colours to not draw attention to yourself) or even not wanting to go to social events that may have an expectation of dressing up, this may indicate you're experiencing changes in the way you see yourself. Finding a few items of clothing that *feel* nice on your skin and boost your confidence, are worth their weight in gold.

4. Photos.

Remove photos and reminders of your pre-cancer body & replace them with *new* ones. Take some updated lovely photos of yourself or have someone else (a friend or photographer) help out, and update your social media and pop them around your home. Having constant reminders of who we were and what we've lost can get in the way of us processing and moving forwards. On dating apps? Update your profile with the new you, using these photos.

5. Quality connections.

Surround yourself with people you can communicate with honestly, that are positive in your life. This is over-simplifying it, but if people bring you down? Don't give them your time. You want relationships with people who contribute to you feeling comfortable, safe and respected. People you can share openly with, to feel supported and loved. Not sure how to know? Notice how you feel after you've spent time with or spoken with people. Do you feel good? Heard? Supported? Or do you notice with some people you walk away feeling drained, misunderstood or judged? Noticing how you feel is a powerful indicator to who you want to spend time with.

6. Treats.

Treat yourself by doing things that help you feel good (helping others, dressing up, exercise, getting a massage, self-pleasure, a bath). You want to experience more 'feeling good' and have that feeling in your life more.

7. Touch.

Connect, have affection, have kisses and skin on skin contact. Hug your friends, hold hands, kiss your partner for the sake of it. Slowly get used to your new body together with a partner and be open about your feelings. If you're with a partner or on a date and feeling shy, or you're not sure where to start, play 'the 2-minute game' or do an 'undressing ritual' for body confidence (detailed in the upcoming section 'simple ideas for connecting'). Touch and intimacy contribute to our mental health and well-being, plus our confidence and self-esteem.

8. Embrace your shy.

You don't have to be naked or full-frontal to have sex, there are ways. You can be intimate with clothes on, lights-off/low or have sex in positions where you're not face to face (which I cover in the 'sexual positions, techniques and tools' section later). Additionally, if *getting* naked is the scary part, the 'undressing ritual' mentioned above is amazing for this. Fear of getting naked in front of a lover/partner/date is common. Think about it, if we're not feeling great about our bodies, it makes sense we feel others won't.

9. Grieve.

Give yourself time to grieve. This is loss. Loss of who we were, and it's okay that you're sad. Allow yourself time to process and be kind to yourself. We lose so much, and we can't move on until we can comfortably say goodbye. It's natural for you to find it difficult to love a different you, but if you find your grief interfering with your life and relationships? Please seek support from a counsellor or psychologist. You don't have to do it alone.

10. Words.

Ask your partner/friends for compliments, but on WHO YOU ARE, *not* how you look. Why? Because if we don't agree, we simply won't agree. Being complimented on you as a person rather than your physical appearance is much more believable, and is the stepping stone towards feeling more confident. And while we're at it, you can ask for compliments in those moments of insecurity. This may seem forced and construed, but it doesn't mean that a compliment is false just because you've reminded someone you'd like to hear one. You're just giving someone permission to offer you flattery in a situation where they may be scared to comment on your appearance or person in any way. It's easier than you think, here's some examples:

How to say it out loud; asking for compliments.
- "I'm feeling a bit low, I'd welcome compliments at the moment."
- "I'm not feeling great, hearing nice things about me might help."
- "I'm feeling pretty self-conscious about my appearance, thoughts?"
- "I'm embarrassed to go out, I feel like I look sick, do I look okay?"

Giving compliments without the beauty focus.
- "I love seeing you smile; it makes me happy."
- "I think you did really well today in conversation."
- "Hearing you laugh gave me so much joy, I think you're amazing."

- "I love you."
- "Everyone was so happy to see you today, you mean a lot to your family/friends/colleagues."
- "I'm so glad you're in my life."
- "You look great in that colour."
- "I love what you're wearing."
- "You're such a great friend."
- "I love our friendship/relationship/connection."
- "You did great today, everyone seemed so happy to see you."
- "You look happy today."
- "Your eyes are shining."
- "I'm perving on your arse right now, do you mind?"

It isn't a cure, but a little love goes a long way!

3.   DATING AND CANCER

Dating is scary, I mean even without a cancer diagnosis. And dropping the 'c-bomb' (saying you've had cancer) on a date can get *really* mixed responses like "but you're normal now, right?". It isn't all that bad, there are some people who are incredibly compassionate and respond with kind curiosity, but how do we find them? How do we actually date again without exhausting ourselves while avoiding all the stress and fear?

1: The filter.

Fatigue and low energy levels are a constant after cancer treatments, even years after. The effort of dating apps, the conversations, the actually going on dates only to be disappointed can all be too much. Here's a pro-tip, literally from dating pro, Georgie Wolf! Say you have or have had cancer *before* the first date. Put things like 'survivor' or whichever words are right for you, on your profile. Mention it in the hello conversation. Additionally, dropping the word 'cancer' may not be the only thing to be nervous about. With varying cancers and their treatments, you may no longer be able to do things like have children or have penetrative sex and knowing when to share these facts can feel daunting. Opening up about these things early on may feel like it will scare some people away (because it will), but this is a good thing because it's a filter. A filter for the people who won't be supportive or understanding, and will waste your time and energy on small talk and dates that go nowhere. You may be reducing the 'pool' so to speak, but a drop in quantity means an *increase in quality*, and this is what we want. Save your precious energy for the actual potentials.

2. Getting naked (or not!).

Our bodies change after cancer, and our confidence and self-esteem can drop. Dating expert Georgie Wolf so insightfully mentions in one of our YouTube video discussions, people can have crippling body image issues from other life-events, not just from cancer, so there are people out there that 'get it'. If you mention you're nervous, people will often respond to that honesty with understanding, as many of us (most of us) have experienced changes in body image at some point. If they don't respond well to you being open and honest? They're not someone you want to be dating.

One way towards getting more confident about getting naked in front of someone is the first step, the filter. You'll be attracting the type of person who will understand if you say you're a bit nervous to show your body.

Another way to work with your body self-consciousness is remembering that you don't need to be naked to get intimate. As previously mentioned, you can wear clothes that cover specific body parts (t-shirts, singlets, teddies, sarongs, towels and more). Plus, you can have the lights low and get intimate in positions that aren't full-frontal (which I go into more detail in the sexual positions section later). This allows you to go slow, not push yourself and reduces that brain-chatter during intimacy. A fun way to reduce the fear of undressing in front of others is in the upcoming section 'simple ideas for connecting'.

3. Warm-up.

I'm not only talking about foreplay, (which is always necessary and will increase your arousal, desire and sexual confidence with others). I'm also talking about warming-up your sexual-*self*-confidence.

- Set yourself a date each week, where you touch your

body softly. All over.

- Get a mirror and look at your body, get to know it, but do so with kindness. If you have scars/replaced or removed body parts, look at other parts of your body first...go slow.
- Wear clothing that makes you *feel* good...if you don't have any, that's okay, buy or borrow some.
- Get a few toys that offer pleasure and stimulation to kickstart your sex and sexual confidence.
- Learning about your body, what it likes and doesn't like is essential for good sex and also, for greater self-confidence. It's an important first step to getting your mojo back.

4. Gamify it.

A little bit of structure goes a loooong way, especially with potentially awkward social environments (that's my nice way of saying dates are pretty awkward).

On a date, you could play a question-and-answer game where you take turns asking and answering questions. I love this as a way to get to know people and 'Q&A' (described in the next section) offers a way to 'rig the conversation' to your favour. By that I mean, after a few rounds of the small talk questions covering topics like food and movie interests, ask the question "what's something that's different about your body?" After they've responded and it's your turn to answer, you can describe your body, but do it in a way of amazement. Like a, 'how amazing is medicine!' kind of framing. It normalises it, shows that you're okay to talk about it and gives them space to ask questions. This is also brilliant as it starts with your date/the other person telling you something strange about their body first, and you listen with curiosity and compassion. It sets the tone.

If getting naked or showing parts of your body feels scary, do an undressing ritual alone or with a date/lover (detailed in the next section 'simple ideas for connecting)'.

If it doesn't go well, you know not to go on another date with them.

5. Baby-stepping towards sex

If you've really hit it off and want to get intimate but are feeling scared, like a broken record I suggest you play the two-minute game (detailed in the next section). I love this game and have been playing it for years including well before, during and after my cancer treatments with partners and also dates. It's brilliant and is the perfect gentle step from enjoying conversation with someone, to enjoying intimacy with someone (without having to leap straight into sex).

6. A trick to 'get into it'

For those times you have a date and you really want to have some sexy-sex, but are a bit nervous if you'll enjoy it or not, I have a trick to help with this. I've mentioned 'arousal' in this book is the 'enjoying' of pleasure. We get hard, wet, hypersensitive skin, our body is flooded with pleasure and happy hormones etc. But, sometimes getting 'into it' can take a bit of time. If you are planning on getting sexy with someone, go for a quick walk beforehand. I kid you not.

A study was actually done to identify the impacts of brief exercise before engaging in sexual activities. It had two groups, one where people had to go for a quick jog and then rate their sexual experience, vs people that didn't exercise and rated their sexual experience (the sexual experience being all watching the same erotic film). Most of the people that went for a jog beforehand reported a much greater experience of pleasure and arousal than those that didn't. It makes sense. Exercise gets blood-flow to your pelvis and deeper genital structures, increasing sensitivity, pleasure, arousal and tissue engorgement. It's so strange, but if you can time your hot-date after your yoga class, or sneak in a brisk walk beforehand, you may have a pretty hot time!

These are just a few ideas and suggestions and I truly hope some of the above has been useful to you. Dating can seem scary, in so many ways, but there are good people out there.

4.   SIMPLE IDEAS FOR CONNECTING

Something we often do, especially in intimacy, is develop patterns. Intimacy, sex, affection can start to look like the same thing, or doing things in a particular and similar way. In regards to rebuilding self-confidence, we need to go slow, maybe change it up so we feel more comfortable and sometimes that's tricky when our relationships and sex look a certain way.

In this section I give you some ways you can have a date-night with someone (or yourself!) which isn't the standard form of what sex might look like to you, but allows you to have fun, connect with yourself, feel good in yourself and feel good with others. The ultimate ideas for ways to reconnect with your body, its pleasure, and really kick-start that confidence process!

The activities I've listed and described are ones I've taught, read about and love to do - and are my top picks for you to try yourself. It's not an exhaustive list, but will give you a start (i.e., trust yourself and you can decide what works for you). Not all will appeal to you, that is fine. They are varied enough so that hopefully there's something for everyone that seems appropriate to try. Remember, these can be done to the level that is right for you, with the person that is right for you. These can be done with a close friend, your carer, by yourself, partners and even family members!

Q&A

I am obsessed with this verbal game and full credit to Roger Butler from Curious Creatures who created it. It's so useful and fun to play if you're in a position where you want to communicate with someone, but it's hard to bring up an awkward topic or start a conversation. It's also great to play any time anywhere, and I love it in social or private settings. It's so simple yet an incredible way to deeply communicate and connect with strangers, loved ones, friends and everyone else. During many of my treatments, I struggled (and still do) to keep up with conversations that involved more than two people as the brain-fog/cancer-brain had my attention span so low. I also struggled at times to have conversations about how I was feeling and where I was at. I often played Q&A as a way to be able to listen to one person at a time, and still have valuable, connective conversations with the people around me. I also play it one-on-one to have meaningful conversations with a partner or friend, while communicating was/is so difficult. Simply put, Q&A makes good conversation great, and when you're struggling, it's a life-saver.

How it works.

Someone asks a question, any question, such as: How was your day? How are you feeling in your body? What do you love about your partner right now? What is your relationship to your sex? Do you like cake more than ice-cream? Anything.

The person sitting to the left of the person who asked the question, answers it first. When they are finished, it goes to the next person to the left, finishing with the person that asked it.

There are a few extra rules:
- Every answer is perfect.
- Every question is perfect.
- No interrupting someone's answer, wait until they have told you they are finished answering, before sharing your thoughts.
- You can 'pass' on a question (or make something up!).

- You can call 'Tangent' or 'Time' by making a 'T' symbol with your hands. This indicates that someone may be off on a tangent or taking too much time to answer. We always say "thank you" for a 'T'.
- The person who asks the question, always answers it last.

It may seem strange, having a verbal Q&A game in a book about connection and the importance of intimacy, but there's a theme here. Cancer interrupts life, which includes relationships. Medications, fatigue, nausea, stress, it all interferes and open communication for some can seem too hard. Try this game, try it a few times, it was and still is, a 'go-to' for me, when I want to connect.

Where? You can play it anywhere. Try it in the bath, the couch, at dinner, in the car, a BBQ or a few rounds at the end of the week to see how you're going. It's a beautiful time to be honest, because the rules are that you can't be interrupted and every answer is perfect.

This is also your saving grace if conversations are hard, paying attention is tricky and keeping up with multiple people talking at once. If you let people know what you need and where you're at, they will most likely help you out. I noticed social chatter was a way for people to let me know that 'everything was fine'. But it wasn't, I couldn't concentrate, I couldn't follow the conversation, I quickly forgot what people were saying and I got super stressed. As soon as I mentioned I needed conversation to slow down, that's exactly what happened. Remember, you will need to let people know what you need, and they will be grateful for the guidance. Q&A is a brilliant way to have social structure, and still offer wonderful connections with everyone present.

Little, lovely treats

Sit down and write a list of 5 - 10 things that are small and easy to do, that make you feel special or connected to yourself. Little, lovely treats. If you have a close friend or loved one, get them to do the same, write a list of little lovely things they enjoy. This could be a foot massage, a bath, a favourite wine, a nice cheese with salami and a childhood film (my personal favourite), moisturising each other's hands/backs/necks/chests, looking at photos together, a blindfolded touch experience, a game of loving Q&A (just described in this section) or dancing to your favourite music.

So, when a time comes, when you're feeling like you would like to connect, be intimate, share affection and don't know what to do? Get the list out and see what you're/you're all in the mood for.

All of these small treats should ideally be things that can be done in your home or very close to where you're staying, and don't take a lot of energy. You want your energy to be spent on connecting and enjoying yourself and others' company, not setting up or travelling to a location.

These 'small treats' lists are your go-to. When you're stuck in your head or having a bad day, get the list out. Soak your feet and moisturise them, do yoga, have a self-pleasure session or pleasure a partner, eat an entire pizza when those taste-buds are back online or get your favourite film and a pot of your favourite tea. The point is that you want an easy way to feel special involving yourself, and possibly those close to you. Simple, sensual, special treats that connect you with yourself/others.

Warming and calming

This small yet intimate task can really let you relax, unwind and get connected. A gentle, beautiful way to connect with yourself or with someone else, is by enjoying a warm bath. Relaxing in a body of warm water (not too hot!) has so many positive effects on the body. Muscles relax, our nervous system down-regulates (relaxes), it can reduce stress, muscle tension eases, pain can lessen, blood circulation improves, the list goes on. Add a cup of tea, a glass of wine, something playing on a screen you can see or some quality Q&A (again see earlier in this section) if you have a 'bath-buddy' with you.

The waterless bath

Baths not your thing, or you don't have one? I have for you, the waterless bath experience. Pop your electric blanket on a nice low setting or warm up a heat pack on the couch and create a warm snuggly cocoon for yourself or for you and your pet, child, friend or lover. The intent is to create warmth, intimacy, safety and connection - baths are not essential for this, but feeling safe and snuggly is.

A royal bathing

Credit for this idea goes to my primary carer, who 'softens' the daily activities to connect and show love, and has also used this technique when caring for a friend while undergoing treatments for brain cancer (spoiler, they loved it!). Is your partner, lover, friend or carer helping you with your personal care? Such as dressing, washing or even simply helping you dry your feet after the shower? If this is the case, every once in a while, ask the person assisting with your care to take their time with it. Turn it into an almost worshipping, lovingly sensual dressing or bathing. Imagine the treatment someone might get in a luxury ancient Roman spa.

Slowly wash the feet, slowly caress and wash the back, take your time enjoying putting clothing on someone, let the materials softly brush over the skin. Attention and intention are drivers of pleasure and going slowly allows this to happen. Yes, we are often time poor and we go into 'automatic mode', however this is a lovely five-minute task which can be added into daily life quite easily and shows care, love and affection. This small activity acts as a reminder to each other, you're not in a clinical environment, you're not a nurse going through the rounds with a patient, you're caring for someone, someone you care about. Be soft, be gentle, be present. What a treat and what a connector. And it only needs to take an extra five minutes or so.

A simple good night kiss

Life is hectic and a cancer diagnosis doesn't lighten the load. Finances, appointments, family life, medications, symptoms and more, can fill up the days. The only time you may actually see a partner or lover is at the end of the day. If this is you, think about taking five minutes, when you're in bed together getting ready for sleep. Lie down facing each other and look into each other's eyes. Touch noses if you like, hold hands, intertwine feet, hold eye contact, share a good-night statement, breathe together or share a kiss on the lips. It's a time where you're both settling down and both in the same spot, it's a great time to use it to connect.

Don't go to bed at the same time as the person you live/share space with? That's okay, ask that you get 'tucked-in' or tuck your partner in. Get the blankets up to their chin, wish them good night, give them a kiss and a few words of love. It's just such a sweet thing. And if you don't share a house with your loved ones? Sweet, loving good night text messages mean the world!

Self-pleasure

Our entire bodies are capable of pleasure and giving yourself some time, some touch and love is a beautiful way to connect with yourself and get those happy chemicals flowing. During treatments you may be tired, stressed, sore, in pain or feeling flat. Whether you're single or partnered, a lovely way to calm and connect with yourself is to give your body, soft, loving touch. This can, but doesn't necessarily need to involve your genitals or you getting aroused. Our bodies are complicated things and treatments can make our body almost feel like a stranger, so getting to know it again can be wonderful.

Give yourself some time, show yourself you're special and set yourself a date. Be it once a fortnight, once a week, or whenever you feel slightly motivated. It's nice, the first few times if you try to leave genitals out of it, just to see what it's like to focus on your body in a different way. We don't give ourselves enough one-on-one time and this is most definitely the case for personal intimate touch. Be curious, explore, hug yourself, scratch, tap, softly touch the skin, find what your body is and isn't enjoying, what it does and doesn't enjoy at that moment. I'm a firm believer that offering ourselves self-pleasure and understanding our bodies is essential for us to be able to connect with others. Regardless if you're partnered or not, having some time with yourself is healthy, it's calming, and it's connecting.

Massage swaps

This may seem like a strange thing to recommend in regards to building body confidence, but hear me out. Touch, care, love and affection are all things many of us forget about during and after treatments. If you're unsure of what your body wants in an arousal, erotic sense, your immediate fallback plan can be massage. Having someone massage you, gives focus on physical, attentive touch without that pressure of it needing to lead to sex. It's pleasurable, it's intimate and gets you connected (and it feels so good!). Massage swaps can also act as an 'ice-breaker', if you're with a partner or on a date and it's been a while since you've touched each other (which is common). This is a lovely and accessible way to ease back into a physical and touch based dynamic without the pressure to 'perform' or 'be sexy'. If you're not partnered and want some touch, but aren't sure how? There are many very skilled professional massage therapists out there, even the 'pop-in' 10-minute massage parlours have amazing touch and anything that connects you to your body and feels good, is a win.

Another amazing benefit of doing massage swaps, is it's a way for a partner or lover to get used to touching your changed body. So often, I support partners through their fear and anxiety of hurting their partner by touching them. A simple massage can be a way to have your partner touch your body and even start to explore areas they are hesitant to touch (like surgery sites or scars). With a little encouragement, direction and permission from you, these fears and anxieties can be overcome, together.

An undressing ritual

How we see ourselves and also, the fear of being naked in front of another person (and ourselves) is one of the most common concerns I help people with. Undressing rituals are a method of removing clothing for yourself, or another, in a way that is gentle while allowing space for nervousness and shyness while inviting acceptance and positive regard. You can do this solo by yourself in front of a mirror as a way to get used to your new body, or with a date or partners.

How it works.

There's a lot of scope for variety here so feel free to bend and change this to suit you, but here's the basics. Standing in front of the mirror or someone else, you choose one item of clothing at a time to take off, and as you remove it you make a personal statement. Something that is true, that is how you feel, but also as a way to process, release and move towards acceptance. It's a neat psychological trick and can be wonderful. If you're doing this with a partner, take turns, so after you remove an item of clothing and make a statement, they do the same. Then it's your turn again, and so on.

<u>By statements I mean things like;</u>

- As I remove my shoe, I let go of how hard I am on myself.
- As I take off my shirt, I let go of my self-consciousness.
- Removing my belt is me removing the restrictions of society's ridiculous beauty standards.
- As I remove my bra, I welcome in love and acceptance of my body.
- As I take off my scarf, I release my fear.
- By taking off my pants, I am freeing myself of anxiety.
- By removing my pink sparkly cowboy hat, I am letting go of my tiring day.

Or, if that form of statement doesn't feel right, you could try positive words as you remove clothing and show parts of your body:

- As I look at my arm, I notice the smooth skin I have.
- While looking into the mirror, I'm loving the freckles I have on my face.
- With my chest exposed I feel an appreciation for being alive.
- As I look at my genitals, I notice the awesome curls in my pubic hair.
- As I see my stomach, I see scars/marks of me living, and making it through
- While looking at my lower back, I like the curve where it joins my bottom.

I have done this by myself in front of a mirror, with a long-term partner and also on a date. It was surprisingly effective on the date, as I was very self-conscious about my body and didn't know how to transition from clothed to well, not-clothed. We both took turns slowly removing an item of clothing, we looked into each-other's eyes, we were honest and it was magic. It helped me relax and it helped them understand how I was feeling and how I was struggling.

Go slow. If you're doing this alone in front of the mirror, it can be quite confronting. Don't feel like you need to fully undress, you may need to do this gradually over time. You could remove one additional item of clothing in the mirror to look at and love each time you do this, so it's nice and slow.

I've done it several times alone, as a way to slowly look at myself and get used to my changed and abnormal body. I cried a lot, but it truly helped me with body acceptance and processing my grief for the body I used to have. Follow yourself, breathe and trust that you can stop if you need to. If you're with someone and you don't want to get naked, you can remove 'imaginary' items of clothing (like an orange feather boa, a sequin vest, rainbow suspenders etc.) or simply ask to stop. You could also do this with someone, where you take turns in removing an item of clothing off of the other person, while making positive statements about their body. Or maybe you choose the item of clothing on yourself to remove and your partner/date shares statements of love and appreciation of that particular body part. The best part of this activity is that there's room to change this to what feels right for you, at the pace that's right for you.

Chatty-massage

If you're liking the ideas in this book about learning more about what you want and giving more feedback in intimacy and pleasure, but aren't really sure how to do that, this one's for you. 'Chatty massage' is very simple, and is the perfect way to get better at figuring out what you want or don't want, and also, how to ask for it. Plus, this is another excellent activity to do, if your partner is feeling a little hesitant to touch your body, because they're scared of hurting you.

How it works.

Easiest done in pairs, one of you is the 'masseuse', and the other receives the 'massage'. But there's a twist. The person lying down, the one receiving the 'massage' is actually directing the masseuse on what to do. Sounds easy right? Well, there's a little more to it.

The person who is receiving direction, the 'masseuse' is only able to do exactly that, receive and follow directions. They cannot take over the experience or offer what they *think* the person receiving might enjoy. They can only follow the directions given by the person lying down who is 'receiving' the massage. The most important part of this however, is that if the masseuse/person following directions doesn't hear something along the lines of "keep going" or "I like this continue please" or a new instruction, they must stop touching the person giving the directions all together by gently removing their hands and waiting for the next instruction.

Why does the person have to stop touching after 10 seconds of silence you ask? For the person who is receiving the directions, this is a lesson in being guided in touch, in taking feedback and more importantly, not making assumptions as to what the other person may want and 'winging it'. For the person receiving the massage/giving directions, it allows them to learn how to ask for what they'd like and how to communicate if they'd like something to stop, continue or to change. It's powerful stuff. It's also an incredible way for them to really explore their body and to learn what they do and don't like at the pace that's right for them.

Giving feedback and knowing how to receive it during intimacy is the thing that makes a good time, a great time. But we're not taught how to talk about sex or our bodies. We're definitely not taught how to explore our likes and dislikes in a safe and compassionate way. The world would be better if we were. Chatty massage (as simple as it seems) is your way to flex those communication muscles and learn so much about your and your partner's pleasure.

If you're not sure where to start, try doing it together sitting on the couch and just on the hand or shoulders to start with. Or have a clothes-on play together while you get used to how it works. You could even set a timer so you have 5 or 10 minutes each of giving and receiving while you're trying it out. You can start by exploring things like soft touch on your arms, maybe scratchy touch on your back, massage touch on your neck and thighs. Soft kisses on your lower back. Feel free to get creative as the person following directions is going to stop if you don't ask for it to keep going, or ask for something to change. This is the safety mechanism, so you both can feel free to relax and have a bit of fun with it.

You may be thinking that the more difficult role in this, is that of the person who's lying down and giving the directions. Funnily enough, when I work with partners together and I teach them this activity it's the complete opposite. It's the person receiving directions and having to stop and withdraw touch after 10 seconds of silence that struggles the most! Due to this, I'm going to repeat the rule as it's surprisingly tough for people, but is so important. If the 'masseuse' doesn't hear a direction after 10 seconds, they must stop what they're doing, remove their hands and wait. This is what will help the person giving direction do exactly that, as they will *have* to give you direction when you stop. So much of our intimacy is guess-work and with the impacts of cancer treatments, clarity and communication could never be more important. Stopping the touch after a short amount of time is a way to help each other practice giving and receiving feedback and most importantly, tuning in to what you do and don't want at the time.

It will 100% feel clunky and awkward at first, just like everything else we try in life for the first time. Don't worry too much about it as this is play, and yes play can be clunky, but it can also be fun. Have a laugh and have another go. Communication is the number one sex move, and this activity is the perfect way to practice.

The two-minute game

Finally we hear about the two-minute game!!!! Life coach Harry Faddis created the 'three-minute game' and I was taught the 'two-minute game' from Roger Butler at Curious

Creatures, and it's simply brilliant. This game is suitable for those experiencing treatment and their loved ones, is great when you have no idea how to connect with someone or where to start and is a wonderful way to gently get to know each other's bodies again.

Here's the rules.
- Set a timer or an alarm on your phone for two minutes.
- Pick who goes first, then that person asks for something they would like for 2 minutes (some examples are listed shortly).
- If you all agree, start the timer and give the person whatever they asked for.
- When the timer goes off, completely stop what you're doing.
- Then it's the next person's turn to ask for something they would like for two minutes.
- If everyone agrees, start the timer and go.
- Once the timer goes off, again, stop what you're doing.
- And repeat.

That's it. Really, that is the game. So simple, yet so

effective. You can play it for as long as you like - 10 minutes or an hour, or however long you have energy and are having fun. Time can really fly when playing this game.

Also, this game can be played with anyone, not just someone you're in a relationship with. It could be a friend, family member, carer and doesn't have to be in pairs. There are so many ways to connect, to touch and be touched, which this game can help you discover.

One of the first (out of possibly hundreds) times I played this, I wasn't sure what to ask for. So, of course, I asked for a shoulder massage. Then, that became a slow back scratch. Then full body soft touch and I was amazed at how starting simply and being left wanting more (thanks to that timer) guided me to what I would like next. Asking for what you want can be difficult at first, but this game allows you to develop that skill with practice. Asking for what we want is such an essential skill to have during cancer treatments (and always).

A common question when introducing the two-minute game in workshops is, "what happens if someone asks for something you don't want to do?" Say "no-thank you" with a smile and discuss an alternative (such as touching the chest or back rather than genitals). It's okay. Wait, it's more than okay, it's wonderful to say 'no'. Saying what we don't want is equally (maybe more) important than saying what we do want. The goal is to find that optimal place where everyone is happy giving and receiving.

Here's a few reasons why this game can work for you:
Our genitals aren't always up for being played with, so when it's your two minutes, ask for something that doesn't include them (you have your whole body).

This game can allow connection, even with different levels of libido. Someone might want sexual touch for two minutes and if you're happy to give it, great! Your two minutes could be something that suits your mood such as "tell me your favourite joke using your hand as a puppet". The possibilities are endless and you can ask for exactly what you want, while easily avoiding what you don't want.

Bodies impacted by treatment can change dramatically and unpredictably, be it sensation, arousal, pain, surgical sites etc. This game allows you to relearn how your body works or doesn't work (where those desensitised parts are, where it's sore, where it's pleasurable, how toys or lubes feel).

If you're playing this with a partner and are worried

about where things may lead to? Take 'typical' sex off the table for the entire game. You could have a 'no genital contact' rule or even leave your clothes on. Remove the pressure to perform or get aroused. Obligation & expectation are the enemy of arousal, feeling safe and relaxed is its catalyst. Get creative, enjoy yourselves without that pressure. You can enjoy pleasure from soft intimate touch anywhere on the body.

The two-minute game has many communication benefits and can act as a gentle ice breaker. With changed sexuality and changed intimacy (with or without illness), can come distance and avoidance. Talking about sex is not easy, especially when things are different. This game gently offers a way to help navigate those tricky feelings while also acknowledging the elephant in the room. While we're at it, let's erase any feelings of 'being selfish' or 'a taker'. Asking for your neck to be gently kissed for two minutes, or to be told why this person loves you for two minutes, is simply playing the game. It can seem difficult, but remember, you have to ask, it's the rules! Through my work as a sexuality and consent workshop facilitator, I'm always shocked at how many people tell me that they have never asked for what they want before. Practice makes perfect and it does get easier the more you do it.

Here's a list of things you could ask for, for your two minutes:

- Can you please lower the lights, put some relaxing music on that I would like, bring me water and join me on the couch in two minutes?
- Hold my hand and tell me how you're doing for two minutes.
- Massage my (insert body part here) for two minutes.
- Starting at my neck, ever so softly touch my entire body, back to feet over two minutes.
- Tell me about your day through interpretive dance.
- Put on a song and show me your silliest/favourite dance move.
- Make me a cup of tea in two minutes.
- I would like to cuddle for two minutes.
- I would like to offer you a shoulder massage for two minutes (that's still your two minutes, but if you're not up for being touched, you can touch others. It's all about what YOU want).
- Massage my head.
- I would like to stroke your hair with your head in

my lap.

- Lightly touch my beautiful bald head for 2 minutes.
- Gently kiss my neck/chest/thighs/back for two minutes.
- Show me how you like to be kissed, for two minutes.
- Kiss my face and tell me things you love about me for two minutes.
- Softly breathe on my entire body, ending with my genitals for two minutes (YUM!).

If you're thinking, "ugh, whatever Tess. Some of us don't know how to just simply know what you want and ask for it." You're right, I hear you. None of us are taught this, but I have a solution for you. A beautiful baby-step towards the 2-minute game and flexing those 'asking' muscles, is by playing the previous activity 'chatty massage'.

Active receiving

'Active receiving' is a way to connect with a lover/partner to the level that is right for you, when you're not feeling sexy or like having sex and maybe need a little bit more time to get those feelings flowing.

It's a one-way touch experience, and a great way to enjoy touch. I'll explain a little more. There are many expectations and misconceptions in intimate activities, and a super common one is that it should always be a two-way experience. You give and receive pleasure at the same time. Well, this doesn't necessarily always have to be the case, and I offer you a wonderful way to connect in a one-way touch format, very similar to 'chatty massage' mentioned previously. This is wonderful for people with mismatched libido, delayed arousal responses (detailed in the 'reactive versus proactive arousal' section in Part 3), if someone is not wanting to receive intimate touch or may not know what they want at that moment, but would love to see a partner have pleasure and enjoy themselves.

How it works.

Someone lies/sits down (or is in any comfortable position), asks for what type of touch they want, and constantly directs that person in how they touch them. The other person does exactly what they are being told to do. That's it! It's incredibly fun and accessible.

Imagine the person giving the touch and receiving the directions has no mind of their own, they are an inanimate object that only responds to commands. For the person following instructions, it can free you from that common brain chatter ("am I doing this right? Are they enjoying this? Are they pretending?"), as you're just doing what you're told.

Some examples of directions the person who is receiving touch (and giving all directions) could give are: "Massage my shoulders. Can you now scratch my back? Yum, thanks, can you go slower and a bit firmer? Softly touch my body up and down, neck to feet with your fingertips and don't stop until I say. Now, lightly pinch my inner thighs. Breathe cool breath on my nipples." Anything you want, just ask.

Unlike in chatty massage where the person following directions stops all together if they don't hear anything after a short while, in 'Active Receiving', the person giving the touch can check in to see if it's how the receiver wants it ("How is this pressure? Would you like me to move my hands faster or slower?") *without* stopping. The person following directions doesn't change anything, doesn't alter any style without being directed. If the person giving touch doesn't receive any directions for a while and isn't sure if this is still what the person receiving still wants? Keep doing what you were last asked to do and ask the question "how could you enjoy this more?"

Similar to chatty massage, this is an incredible skill to learn in the bedroom. Giving directions, asking for what we want, checking in with a lover to get feedback on their level of enjoyment, communicating your desires, all of this leads to better communication and better sex. If you get tired? Simply stop the activity whenever one of you wants. The goal is to enjoy receiving and to enjoy giving. 1 minute, 10 minutes, 20 minutes, it's all perfect.

If you're unsure, give it a go, clothes on, on the couch, using just an arm or hand. Practice following directions, practice giving directions, practice checking in and identifying what you want. There is no goal here, just to have a touch experience, to give or receive pleasure, and enjoy connecting with a partner. It may feel clunky at first, but with practice it flows very easily and you will be amazed at how much you learn about your partner and their body (and yours!).

If this sounds like fun to you, but asking for what you want and giving directions seems a bit daunting, or taking directions and not being the one driving the experience sounds tough, I recommend playing 'chatty massage' or the

'2-minute game' a few times first, before jumping into this activity. I say this only because it won't be enjoyable if you're still getting used to these styles of intimate communication. Those two activities are wonderful (and fun!) ways to develop these amazing sexy skills.

5. SEXUAL POSITIONS, TECHNIQUES & TOOLS

Sex as a functional activity is extremely adaptable, with so many possible positions we can put our bodies in and so many adaptations to suit our needs. Here, I offer some suggestions and ways to alter the positions of your body, to get around body confidence concerns.

Explore, experiment, but make sure you do it from a place of communication and curiosity. You all want to be comfortable and, most importantly, safe, so have a chat beforehand with your lover. Treat it like a brainstorm, note what parts of your body you're nervous about showing and figure out how to work around them comfortably and safely. It mightn't seem 'sexy' at first, but these conversations will get easier, and it will make things *much* better. And remember, if it's good, you'll want it more.

Positions for self-consciousness

As discussed previously our bodies change and so is the way we see ourselves, which can interfere with our sex. Talking about it, is the number one approach with this to explain how you're feeling. I spoke with a husband and wife recently and she told me she had refused to get naked in front of her husband for the entire time since cancer diagnosis from self-consciousness (a period of years). She regrets it now as they have spoken about it since, and all he wanted was to hold his partner and love her. Even just naming the elephant in the room can be such a relief, and then thinking about other options can come.

Wearing clothes/lingerie during sex if you're not wanting to be completely naked is a simple method to ease self-consciousness. There's no shame in wearing a t-shirt during sex, nor a skirt/sarong wrapped around the waist. If you're not ready to look into your lovers' eyes during sex? Try the side-lying position which is like a 'spoon', or someone being taken from behind, or even sitting on your partner's lap/being sat on, with the person on top facing away. You could also, under the covers, self-pleasure yourselves, but together, or offer pleasurable touch to each other while under the covers and the lights low. This is still sex.

Positions for stomas and catheters

Attention! Sex is still possible if you have a stoma bag/pouch or catheter, even if you're feeling a little hesitant or shy to give it a go.

For stomas, a helpful tip is to empty the pouch before you start and there are smaller pouches which can be worn for 'intimate moments'. Positioning yourself or your lover to reduce the risk of pressure on the pouch is helpful. The standard missionary position can be fine, if the person on top has the upper body strength to hold themselves up. Other positions, such as playing with someone from behind or standing up while someone is lying on the edge of the bed or chair can work well to avoid bumping and putting pressure on the pouch. The spooning position is also wonderful for people with stoma pouches and catheters, as the person in the front has more space in front of them. There are many, well-designed intimate-wear options for all genders, for those who have stoma pouches/appliances and are self-conscious about it showing.

For catheters, before any sexual activity, emptying the urine collection device and securing it out of the way is recommended. For those with a penis, you can fold the catheter tube down the penis shaft and cover your penis and tube together with a condom, which holds them together in place and penetration is still very achievable. Just make sure you have enough spare tube at the top for your erection to grow/penis to expand with blood-flow and afterwards, wash and secure it back in place. For those with a vulva, taping the catheter tube out of the way on the abdomen/thigh keeps it out of the way. Having a wash afterwards is recommended (to avoid UTIs) and securing it back in place.

If you want to stop, then stop. Remember, don't force it, don't put up with pain, self-pleasure is always there for a partner if someone wants to continue. Hey, if you stop sex as it's a bit too difficult or is no longer pleasurable and your lover wants to continue pleasure through touching themselves? Offer them a hand!

It's important to note, bodies are complicated and what might work one day, might not the next. It's okay, it's normal, but you need to communicate how you're doing during and after sex, such as telling your lover that you're getting self-conscious, or you want to change position. Comments like this, are you being great at sex. Make the adjustments you need, see if everyone is doing okay, keep going if you're all comfortable and check in after.

How to say it out loud.

- "Can we please pause for a second? I just need to re-adjust these cushions, thanks!"
- "I'd love to keep going, but we may need to brainstorm a new position as I'm in my head/self conscious…"
- "I'm really loving this, could we slow down a bit?"
- "Can you pass that T-shirt quickly? I want to keep going, but just want to cover my chest up so I can be more present."
- "I may need to stop; would you like to continue with self-pleasure? Would you like me to touch your body while you pleasure yourself?"
- "Can we please pause? I'm feeling a bit odd and need a moment, thank you."
- "I don't want to keep going as we are, but really want to continue being intimate with you. Is there some form of different touch or pleasure you might enjoy that I can offer you?"
- "Just letting you know everything is great, I'd just like to keep the lights-low, thanks!"
- "How could you/we enjoy this more?"
- "Is there a speed or pressure of touch that you might enjoy more?"

- "How could this be even better for both of us?"
- "I just wanted to check in, are you comfortable?"
- "Please let me know if you need to change positions at any time."
- "I'm loving connecting with you, I just want to make sure you're comfortable?"
- "I know I'm not moving much, but I'm really enjoying this and I'd like to keep going."

Communicating after intimacy (aftercare).
- Thank you so much, that was wonderful. Is there anything you need or would like in this moment?
- Can we please cuddle for a while? I'd like to stay connected with you for a bit longer.
- I'd love to know what you enjoyed about that experience, and I'll share the same.
- I'd love to know if there was anything you might like to do differently next time, or explore more, and I'll share the same.
- Can we lie here together while I catch my breath?
- This has brought up a few emotions, I'm okay, but chatting for a short while would be lovely.

6. TIPS FOR LOVED ONES

Seeing a loved one go through cancer is tough, and so can knowing what to say or how to act. Whether you're a carer, friend, family member or partner, there are ways to offer connection without overstepping a line. And don't worry, we won't break!

People undergoing treatments can be seen as easily hurt, fragile or dangerous, and rightly so. There are many side-effects of treatments, some of them are mental and some of them are physical. However, let's remember this: connection is always important, and even if someone's body and mind are changing, there are still ways to be there with someone.

Understandably it can be hard to know what to do. It's also normal, when seeing a loved one be so unwell, to want to avoid causing any other harm and through that, create physical distance. That might look like reducing touch and physical contact, or even like possible avoidance. If you're a partner, lover, friend or carer of someone during treatment, I implore you, I beg you, to offer them touch. Treatment is damaging and also detaching, and that distance feeds into our low self-esteem and low body-confidence. We need the treatment, yes, but we also need care, to feel connected to ourselves and to those around us. Don't be afraid of us, be cautious and curious with us. Think of it as getting into 'ask first' mode.

For simple touch, a peck on the lips or cheek? It's okay! We are not radioactive, we won't give you cancer and we won't break, if we all just take a little care. How do we know what to do or what not to do? We ask.

How to say it out loud.

- "Would you like me to take your hand?"
- "Is there any way you might like some loving/comforting touch right now?"
- "Would you like a hug?"
- "I'd love a cuddle; how does that sound to you?"
- "I'd love to connect with you, are there any sore spots I should avoid if I went in for a cuddle?"
- "I'd love to connect with you right now, is there a form of touch you would like?" (Arm around the shoulder, hand holding, hug from behind, foot massage and more.)
- "I love you and want to offer you affection, is there anything that would comfort you at the moment?"

- "I miss you, but I'm worried I'll hurt you if I squeeze you too hard. Is there a way I can snuggle into you?"
- "I'm wanting to show you love and affection, such as a kiss on the lips or cheek, how do you feel about that?"
- "I'm checking you out right now, fancy a kiss?"

If you're being made an offer of connection and it's not a good time? I offer some examples shortly on ways to navigate that, however a simple, "thank you, but I'm not quite up for it at the moment" is perfect. Even if the person receiving this offer is not up for it right then, you're showing love, care, concern for their well-being and the desire to remain connected. It means the world.

Not in the mood?

Whether you're the person with cancer or the partner of, there will be times when you don't feel like being intimate with others, that is fine, that is normal, that is understandable. There will also be times when you feel like connecting somehow, but aren't sure how. There are lots of places to start: Get in the bath and relax or wrap yourself in blankets with a hot-water bottle, maybe touch your body, snuggle a pet with your favourite film, ask the person you're with to intertwine your legs while you both sit on the couch or lean into their chest. During treatments, you're not going to want intimacy or touch all of the time, so feel free to let loved ones know how you're feeling and speak up in the moments it seems plausible. If you do receive an offer of intimacy and connection and you're not up for it? Remember, that's okay, that's fine, that's normal. But also remember to say thanks for the offer and be kind when you say no thanks, because you want the offers to keep coming!

How to say it out loud.

- "Thank you, that sounds amazing, it's not the best moment, can we see how I'm going later?" (Or tomorrow, or after lunch)
- "Thanks, I'm feeling quite nauseous/tired/some pain, for the moment I need to sit still, can we maybe connect later or another day?"
- "I'm really not feeling well, I'd like to sit alone for a while. Thank you so much for offering a cuddle, rain-check?"

- "I'd love to kiss you, but my mouth is a bit sore at the moment, would you like some soft neck touch instead?"
- "Yes, I'd love a hug! But just letting you know I'm not up for much else, thank you!."
- "I don't think I'm up for a hug right now, would you like to hold my hand?"
- "I'm pretty low on energy at the moment, but something soft and gentle would be lovely, like a snuggle?"
- Or if you're ADHD and ridiculously blunt like me "Thanks for the offer of a kiss, I'm currently trying not to vomit in my mouth, so will need to rain-check" (we both had a giggle at that).

To those undergoing treatments, if you feel your partner/lover/friend is avoiding you, unattracted to you and doesn't want to touch you? They may just be thinking they are protecting you, avoiding potentially hurting you or feel like they're pestering/pressuring you, so are pulling away. Be the one to communicate and offer a connection. Offer to snuggle, offer to touch their back while they're standing next to you, ask for a long hug hello, it guides them, and can lead to further connections. It meant the world to me, having my hand held and legs entwined on the couch with a cup of tea and chats. It was meaningful and intimate, that at times was my sex. Simple things like that were so important, and I know is/was to others during treatments.

7. FOR MY FELLOW RAINBOW-FLAGGERS

For people in the LGBTQIA+ community, medical institutions can be very difficult. I remember sitting in the chemo-chair with my then partner holding my hand. The nurse approached and looked at us holding hands, then looking at her said "oh, isn't that sweet you're such good *friends*". I know the nurse meant well, but it was devaluing to me and my partner. I did not feel like I was seen as a person, nor my partner respected. I also did not have the energy to continually educate everyone around me all day every day and advocate for who I am and for others. It's exhausting and with cancer, I didn't have it in me. So, I withdrew and I became reluctant to share my personal story with most clinicians. This is particularly important for people with cancers such as prostate, testicular, cervix, ovaries or breast (just to name a few), as these cancers are *very* gendered. Due to this people can isolate themselves from the supports that are out there they may feel unwelcome or unseen. Speaking personally, the 'sisterhood' is very strong in breast cancer and as a non-binary person, was difficult to ignore. I avoided so many (pretty much all) support networks due to this as I did not feel welcome. If you're someone who resonates with this, if you belong to communities that are marginalised, I ask you to reach out. Reach out to that one person on your treating team you can have an honest, non-shaming conversation with. Reach out to the nurse asking for any resources the hospital knows of that are accessible and inclusive. Reach out to a friend, to find a cancer support group near you or online that is gender aware, recognises pronouns, alternative relationship models, and partnerships that are not only heterosexual. They are out there, but you may need help finding them. Feeling safe and supported is everything.

RESOURCES

Because there's limited work on sexuality and cancer and well, actual realistic and accessible sexuality education in general, resources can be hard to find. So, here are some, of varied mediums depending on what suits you best.

The 'A Better Normal' mini-book series
Available globally on Amazon in paperback or eBook format, you can search by author 'Tess Devèze' or by book title.

If you're needing support, practical solutions and guidance on more specific side-effects, or looking for help regarding a specific treatment, the 'A Better Normal' mini-book series covers quite a range.

Books in the 'A Better Normal' mini-book series are:
- 'A Better Normal for **Libido**; Your Guide to Rediscovering Intimacy After Cancer'
- 'A Better Normal for **Vaginal Dryness & Pain**; Your Guide to Rediscovering Intimacy After Cancer'
- 'A Better Normal for **Body Confidence**; Your Guide to Rediscovering Intimacy After Cancer'

- 'A Better Normal for **Chemotherapy**; Your Guide to Rediscovering Intimacy After Cancer'
- 'A Better Normal for **Hormone Therapy**; Your Guide to Rediscovering Intimacy After Cancer'
- 'A Better Normal for **Fatigue**; Your Guide to Rediscovering Intimacy After Cancer'
- 'A Better Normal for **Changes in Erection**; Your Guide to Rediscovering Intimacy After Cancer'
- 'A Better Normal for **Radiotherapy**; Your Guide to Rediscovering Intimacy After Cancer'
- 'A Better Normal for **Pain**; Your Guide to Rediscovering Intimacy After Cancer'

The all-in-one resource, 'A Better Normal; Your Guide to Rediscovering Intimacy After Cancer'

Available globally on Amazon in paperback or eBook, you can search via author 'Tess Devèze' or by book title.

If you liked the information in this book, but feel you need guidance on more, the book 'A Better Normal; Your Guide to Rediscovering Intimacy After Cancer' has all of the information included in the entire mini-book series and more. It's your one stop shop for everything you need to know about sexuality and cancer, in the one book.

Vulva Pleasure Masterclass

(connectable.podia.com/vulva-masterclass)

For anyone with a vulva who is experiencing pain and dryness, or is experiencing loss of sensation, pleasure, arousal and orgasm. This online Masterclass teaches vulva massage, which can be done on yourself or with a partner. Through massage and neurological concepts, things like arousal and pleasure can be recovered while helping heal tissues through increasing blood-flow with massage. This Masterclass is also suitable for people with vaginismus and vulvodynia.

Penis Pleasure Masterclass

(connectable.podia.com/penis-pleasure)

For anyone with a penis who is experiencing changes in erection and orgasm, or is experiencing loss of sensation, function and pleasure. This online Masterclass teaches soft penis massage, which can be done on yourself or with a partner. Through massage and neurological concepts, things like sensation and pleasure can be recovered while helping recover erectile function through increasing blood-flow with massage. This Masterclass is particularly beneficial for people post prostatectomy.

A libido and intimacy recovery program for couples

'Connection & Cancer: Reclaim Your Intimacy & Desire'.
(connectable.podia.com/libido-after-cancer)

If you would like personal support through the exact process of *how* to recover your pleasure, intimacy and libido, then this is for you. It's with me online guiding you every step of the way, and is done in the privacy of your own home. Filled with information, fun and practical solutions that I take you through for libido recovery. The people who I've worked with in this program are having life-changing results. It's an absolute honour to guide people to recover what they felt was lost forever.

'ConnectAble Therapies' (connectabletherapies.com)
For consultations and further resources on sex, intimacy & cancer.

Facebook global support group: *'Intimacy and Cancer'.* This group is for any cancer, any gender and is a very supportive space.

Instagram '@connectable_therapies', where I regularly share helpful information.

YouTube Channel on sex, intimacy & cancer: type *"Intimacy and Cancer CHANNEL"* to find it.

If you prefer video formats over reading (as cancer-brain & reading don't go well together), this YouTube Channel is filled with short videos discussing all things sex, intimacy and cancer.

'ConnectAble Courses' (connectable.podia.com)

A site of intimacy and cancer online courses for sexual recovery. Including the Masterclasses, libido recovery program and webinar mentioned here.

Intimacy & Cancer Information Webinar

(connectable.podia.com/webinar-intimacyaftercancer)

A free information webinar discussing the impacts cancer treatments have on intimacy and sexuality. It has a particular focus on libido and how it can be recovered.

Other amazing resources:

'A Touchy Subject' (atouchysubject.com)

For people with prostate cancer or experiencing changes in erection. Victoria Cullen is *the* person to go to, about sexuality and intimacy post a prostate cancer diagnosis. She also has a YouTube channel and through her website access to free resources and rehabilitation programs.

'The Art of The Hook Up' (artofthehookup.com)

This site from dating expert and communication extraordinaire is by Georgie Wolf. Not cancer specific, but incredibly on-point and with relative information for anyone struggling with the dating scene. She has podcasts, blogs, eBooks and more. She's also a workshop facilitator and a bit of a superstar here in Australia!

'Curious Creatures' (curiouscreatures.biz)

For online workshops and much more education on self-development and sexuality. They provide articles, podcasts and streamable workshops which are all very practical and very accessible. I have the privilege to work for this company, their work is changing lives.

'Bump'n Joystick' (getbumpn.com)

An intimacy aid designed for people with impaired upper limb and fine-motor function. Suitable for all genders and is flexible to varied body shapes. This toy was designed by the global disability and OT community, and it's pretty incredible.

'The Ziggy' (luddi.co)

Another intimacy aid designed for people with limited upper limb and intact fine-motor function. Designed by the disability community and healthcare professionals, this is a multi-purpose vibrator for all genders. It's also able to be used while in a wheelchair, so is a wonderfully accessible item.

Pelvic and sexual health osteopath

For those who live in Melbourne, Australia, we have one of the top pelvic health osteopaths you'll ever find. Dr Andrew Carr from the *'Whole Being Health Collective'* is referred to as *'the body whisperer'* in clinical and sexual health circles. He works with the entire body, however has expertise and clinical focus on pelvic and sexual health. In particular, people experiencing pelvic pain including after treatments, vaginismus, atrophy and is trauma informed.

If you're not located in Melbourne, there are pelvic floor osteopaths, physiotherapists and OTs all over the world. Simply search online "Pelvic floor osteopath/physio/OT (insert the name of your city/town here)". You'll find someone near you.

Support groups in your area

If you search in google "Cancer Support (insert city/town where you live here)", there should be a list of businesses and companies that have programs near you. Some online or in person. They mightn't be sexuality specific, but there is always opportunity for discussions and learning.

ACKNOWLEDGEMENTS

For anyone and everyone out there affected by cancer, this book is for you. There can be so much to consider, to have to endure, to have to keep track of, that many parts of life take a back seat. Thank you for caring about your intimacy and connections during such a time, be it connections with yourself or with others. I hope you're supported and I truly hope there is something in this book for you.

I'm forever grateful to my clients and the thousands I support online who so openly and vulnerably share their struggles, and also their triumphs with me. This book would not exist without you. I'm inspired and amazed by you all, daily.

Thank you, to my partners and carers over the years Rog, Robi and Kane, my family and my global network of friends. There were some very dark places during treatments and you all got me through. To my booby buddies (my breast care nurses) Claire & Monique, you're my angels. Ricky Dick my oncologist - you're simply the best (Tina Turner style!) and to my RADelaidies.

Lastly, to acknowledge the incredible ethics, values and

approaches to sexuality and communication from Roger Butler at Curious Creatures (and their generosity with sharing their content with me), the occupational therapy & sexuality community (yeah OT-siggers!) and the revolutionary perspectives and therapeutic trainings I received from Deej & Uma, at the Institute of Somatic Sexology (ISS).

ABOUT THE AUTHOR

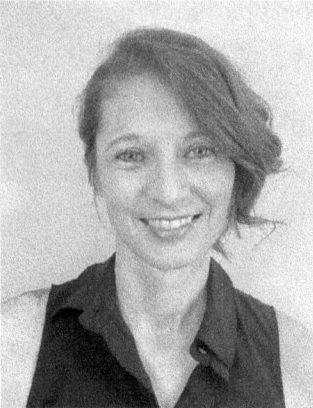

Tess Devèze is an occupational therapist (OT) having completed their bachelor degree in Melbourne Australia, founding ConnectAble Therapies, a community sexuality OT and sexology clinic focussing on sexuality and intimacy for people with neurological conditions, cancer, chronic illness and disability. They have also completed certification and trainings via the Institute of Somatic Sexology. Alongside being a sexuality OT, Tess is also a sexuality educator & workshop facilitator, and has facilitated and educated thousands of people in the topics of communication, consent, sexuality, pleasure and relationship dynamics for nearing a decade. Tess founded the global online initiative 'Intimacy and Cancer', an online support space for people of all cancers and genders to access sexual support.

As a non-binary, queer, disabled person living with cancer, Tess's work is inclusive and advocates for sexual rights for disabled, neurodivergent, gender queer/diverse and LGBTQIA+, communities, which they proudly belong to.

Tess was diagnosed with stage 3 breast cancer at the age of 36 and is still undergoing treatments.

Find them at www.connectabletherapies.com

DID YOU ENJOY THE BOOK?

As an independent author, my work survives through your support. There are so many people affected by cancer, suffering in silence. With each review or word-of-mouth recommendation you make, we can reach the many out there who are struggling and need support.

Please leave a review by visiting where you purchased this book. It's just 1 minute of your time, but could be the thing that helps this reach someone who needs it, someone who needs a better normal too.

Got feedback? Please leave a review! Plus, I'd love to hear from you. You can reach me via email at tess@connectabletherapies.com or via Instagram @connectable_therapies.

www.ingramcontent.com/pod-product-compliance
Lightning Source LLC
Chambersburg PA
CBHW062149020426
42334CB00020B/2555